The Hypothyroidism Handbook:

BY LINDSEY P

An Everyday Guide to Natural Solutions of living with Hypothyroidism including increased energy, lasting weight loss, and general well-being

2nd Edition

Table of Contents

Introduction

I want to thank you and congratulate you for purchasing the book, "The Hypothyroidism Handbook: An Everyday Guide to Natural solutions of living with Hypothyroidism including increased energy, lasting weight loss and general well-being".

This book contains proven steps and strategies on how to treat Hypothyroidism naturally. Hypothyroidism is known as the condition where in one has an abnormally low production of thyroid hormones. Lacks of thyroid hormones affect the body in many ways, such as:

- An enlarged heart

- Having a hard time losing weight which leads to too much weight gain

- Worsening heart failure

- Accumulation of fluid in the lungs which can lead to many respiratory diseases

With the help of this book, you will get to know the signs and symptoms of Hypothyroidism, its causes, and the various natural ways that you can combat the disease. If you want to live a long and healthy life without Hypothyroidism, you have to start reading this book now.

Thanks again for purchasing this book, I hope you enjoy it!

Chapter 1: What is Hypothyroidism?

Hypothyroidism is a medical condition characterized by a disorder in the endocrine system which causes the thyroid gland to be unable to produce sufficient thyroid hormones known as thyroxine (T4) and triodothyronine (T3). The signs and symptoms are varied and in some children, symptoms are not palpable at all especially if the case is only mild. In severe cases, however, hypothyroidism can delay the growth and intellectual development of the child causing severe medical condition known as cretinism. When suspected, the method used for diagnosis is through a series of blood tests that measure the thyroxine levels in the blood and the thyroid stimulating hormone (TSH).

The most common cause of hypothyroidism is insufficient supply of iodine in the diet. This situation is fairly common worldwide. In countries with enough dietary iodine though, the common cause of hypothyroidism is the condition known as Hashimoto's Thyroiditis, an auto-immune medical condition wherein the body's own immune cells destroy and attack the thyroid gland. There are other possible causes of hypothyroidism including injury to the hypothalamic area of the brain, history on radioactive iodine treatment, injury to the anterior pituitary gland, inborn thyroid malfunction, medications and history of thyroid surgery.

Hypothyroidism can also cause other disorders that directly or indirectly affect the thyroid gland. Since thyroid hormones affect mental development, cellular processes and growth, the insufficient production of thyroid hormones can bring a widespread abnormality in the body's internal processes.

Hypothyroidism can certainly be treated but it could require a lifelong medication. A dose of manufactured L-thyroxine is enough to bring back the levels of TSH or thyroid-stimulating hormones in normal levels. Dosage varies according to the symptoms and level of hormones lacking. Medications, however, can last a lifetime with the exception of other pre-conceived conditions.

Hypothyroidism is fairly common in adults. It affects 3-5% of the adult population. It is more common in women and the risks increase with advancing age. Interestingly, hypothyroidism does not only appear in humans. Dogs and cats are also susceptible in acquiring this disorder.

What are thyroid hormones and why are they important?

The thyroid gland produces thyroid hormones. This gland is situated right below the Adam's apple in men and generally on the lower part of the neck for women and children (just above the collar bones). Thyroid gland is wrapped around the trachea (windpipe) and is shaped like a butterfly. It has two lobes (wings) attached by an isthmus (the middle part).

Iodine is important because the thyroid gland uses this to fuel its functions. Iodine is present commonly in a person's diet including salt, bread and sea foods. Thyroxine (T4) makes up the 99% of thyroid hormones while triodothyronine (T3) accounts for only 1%. T3, however, has the most biological importance because it affects more biological activity. When released into the bloodstream, T4 is converted to T3 in response to the demands for active hormones that affect cell metabolism.

How are thyroid hormones regulated?

There is a chain of command being followed in the regulation of thyroid hormones. It is not surprising because the human body is governed by different internal processes. The thyroid is regulated by the pituitary gland, which is another gland located in the brain. Similarly, the pituitary gland is regulated by the thyroid gland in a 'feedback' effect of thyroid hormones. Both glands are then regulated by the hypothalamus, another important gland in the brain.

The hypothalamus releases thyrotropin (TRH) which signals the pituitary gland to release the thyroid-stimulating hormones (TSH). Once TSH is released in the bloodstream, the thyroid gland will then release thyroid hormones that are known as T3 and T4. If there are any disruptions, then these result to insufficient supply of thyroid hormones and bring about the condition called hypothyroidism.

The pituitary gland controls thyroid hormone production. As a result, if there's insufficient supply of thyroid hormone circulating in the bloodstream, the pituitary gland will attempt to balance the insufficiency by producing more thyroid-stimulating hormones (TSH). This to stimulate more thyroid hormone production and normalize cell growth. In contrast, if there is an excessive amount of thyroid hormones in the blood, the pituitary gland will decrease the production of TSH to lower the production of thyroid hormones.

Chapter 2: Causes, Signs and Symptoms of Hypothyroidism

Before you get to know what could be done to fight off the disease, you should first get to know what causes it in the first place. There are numerous causes of hypothyroidism. The primary and the most common cause of this illness is the inadequate functioning of the thyroid gland itself. Another cause may also be the insufficient stimulation of the TSH or thyroid-stimulating hormones. This is also referred to as the central hypothyroidism. Primary hypothyroidism in turn is a result of iodine deficiency which also accounts for most cases of goiter worldwide. Both primary and central hypothyroidism are caused by other underlying factors that are discussed below.

- **Pregnancy.** When women are pregnant or in that span of time just after giving birth, they tend to produce antibodies courtesy of their thyroid glands and that's why thyroid hormone production is lessened. The rise of blood pressure while pregnant may cause a miscarriage to happen or may affect the fetus.

- **Autoimmune Diseases**. Those who suffer from autoimmune diseases such as Hashimoto's Thyroiditis is more likely to develop Hypothyroidism as their immune system is not working properly to protect them.

- **Radiation Therapy**. If you are already suffering from cancers of the neck and head that require

9

radiation to be treated, you may also get to suffer from Hypothyroidism in the future.

- **Thyroid Surgery**. Of course, surgeries involving the thyroid can be big causes of Hypothyroidism because it halts or diminishes Thyroid Production.

- **Medication**. There are certain types of medicine that causes Hypothyroidism, especially those that are used to treat Psychiatric diseases such as Lithium. It would be best for you to ask your doctor about the certain effects of the medicines that you take in. Drugs used to treat hyperthyroidism can result to hypothyroidism. These include methimazole, propylthiouracil, lithium, psychiatric medication, amiodarone and potassium iodide.

- **Pituitary injury.** Sometimes, the Pituitary gland fails to produce the sufficient number of Thyroid Stimulating Hormones or TSH because there are benign tumors in the Pituitary Gland. These then cause Hypothyroidism to happen. This may occur when there is an insufficient supply of blood in the area or as a result of a brain surgery. If the pituitary gland is injured, then there is a considerable amount of TSH lacking in the bloodstream. Consequently, if there is a low level of TSH in the blood, the thyroid gland will not be able to offer adequate supply of thyroid hormones. Hypothyroidism associated with pituitary gland injury may also lead to other conjunctive hormone deficiencies since the pituitary gland also regulates other processes such as reproduction, adrenal functions and growth.

- **Congenital Diseases.** Some babies are born with defective thyroid glands or no thyroid glands at all. It may be a cause of problems during pregnancy or because their parents also have Hypothyroidism.

- **Severe Iodine Deficiency.** You know why they say that you have to eat foods that are rich in Iodine? Well, it's because Iodine Deficiency causes a lot of diseases such as Goiter and in this case, Hypothyroidism. In some parts of the world where people do not get enough supply of iodine in their diets, hypothyroidism accounts for 5-15% of the population. These areas include India, Chile, Zaire and Ecuador. Remote mountain areas such as the Himalayas and the Andes mountain ranges have the most severe cases of hypothyroidism. In the United States, however, this condition became rare since the inclusion of iodine in their salt and bread. **Thyroid gland disease:** This means that the thyroid gland is unable to produce or release enough thyroid hormones and so the pituitary gland releases more TSH or thyroid-stimulating hormone in an attempt to stimulate the thyroid gland to produce more thyroid hormones. As a result, TSH levels in the blood are significantly high while thyroid hormones T3 and T4 are considerably low.

- **Hashimoto's Thyroiditis**: This type of disease or condition is the most common cause of hypothyroidism in the United States. This is coined after Dr. Hakaru Hashimoto who discovered this condition in 1912. In this condition, the thyroid gland is usually enlarged (a condition characteristically known as goiter) and is unable to produce thyroid hormones. This is a type of auto-immune disease wherein the immune cells attack and destroy the thyroid tissues. It is believed to be hereditary and is more common in women. This type of condition also brings forth other auto-immune diseases such as diabetes and pernicious anemia.

- **Pituitary or hypothalamic disease**: In cases where the thyroid gland is normal, T3 and T4 produced and released in the blood are still not indicative of normal thyroid hormone levels. If the pituitary and the hypothalamic glands are not functioning properly, the T3 and T4 production is still affected even if the thyroid gland is functional. Pituitary disease causes secondary hypothyroidism and hypothalamic gland disease causes tertiary hypothyroidism.

- **Lymphocytic Thyroiditis**: This is a condition where inflammation of the thyroid gland is caused by a particular white blood cell known as lymphocyte. This is common after pregnancy and 8% of women are affected after giving birth. In this case, hyperthyroid (excessive amount of thyroid hormone leaked out from enflamed gland) phase occurs first followed by a period of 6 months under hypothyroid phase. After 6 months or so, these women return to normal thyroid functioning although in some cases, hypothyroid phase is prolonged.

- **Thyroid destruction due to radioactive iodine surgery**: Patients who have a history of hypothyroid treatment using radioactive iodine surgery are often left with little or no thyroid tissue at all after surgery. This may have been caused by the dosage of iodine given and the size of the pituitary gland itself after surgery. If there is no recorded activity on the thyroid area after 6 months, it can be concluded that the thyroid gland will no longer perform adequately.

Common Symptoms of Hypothyroidism:

Signs and symptoms of hypothyroidism are often subtle. This condition is fairly common but the signs and symptoms can either be mild or severe. There are numerous signs and symptoms associated with hypothyroidism that may or may not directly be a cause of underlying insufficiency in thyroid hormones. In countries where there is enough supply of iodine in the diet, for example, Hashimoto's Thyroiditis produces the mass effect of a goiter. In severe cases though, hypothyroidism or medically known as myxedema could possibly lead to coma and death.

The insufficient supply of thyroid hormones in the body is conclusive to an underactive thyroid gland. As a result, the organs and internal processes are affected causing emotional, mental and physical symptoms. The following signs and symptoms are only visible in adults.

Signs:

- Cold extremities

- Carpal Tunnel Syndrome – a median entrapment neuropathy which causes numbness, pain, paresthesia (sensation of tingling or tickling feeling) and other symptoms associated with the distribution of the median nerve. This is primarily because of the underlying cause which is the compression of these median nerves at the wrist in the carpal tunnel.

- Dry and coarse skin

- Myxedema – it is a severe case of hypothyroidism characterized by a deposition of mucopolysaccharides in the dermis (inner layer of the skin).

- Slow Pulse rate

- Hair loss

- Peripheral Edema (abnormal accumulation of fluid)

- Delayed relaxation of tendon reflexes (slow reflex) – this is diagnosed after an ankle jerk reflex which is a characteristic sign of hypothyroidism. It also correlates with the severity level of the thyroid hormone deficit.

- Serious cavity effusions including but not limited to pericardial, ascites and pleural effusions

Symptoms:

- Constipation

- Feeling cold

- Weight gain but interestingly with poor appetite

- Poor memory and lack of concentration

- Fatigue

- Hoarse voice

- Shortness of breath

- Poor hearing condition

- Paresthesia – also means a tickling, tingling, prickling, pricking and burning sensation on the skin with no long-term apparent effects.

- Menorrhagia – this is also known as Hematomunia which is characterized by abnormally heavy and prolonged menstrual periods over a regular interval.

- Oligomenorrhea – infrequent menstruation

Advanced cases of hypothyroidism may exhibit other symptoms such as slurred and slow speech, decreased sensations (taste and smell), sleepiness, low sex drive due to decreased libido, puffiness of hands, face and feet and depression.

Myxedema Coma:

This is a rare condition but it is certainly a life-threatening state of severe hypothyroidism. This usually occurs to people with hypothyroidism who also acquired another type of illness. It can also be the first representation of hypothyroidism. Signs and symptoms include decreased body temperature in the absence of shivering, slow heart rate, altered consciousness level and reduced respiratory effort. Skin changes and swelling of the tongue may also be indicative of this condition.

Hypothyroidism in children:

Hypothyroidism in children is not common; and often, the signs and symptoms are very mild to not being obvious at all. In some cases, however, these signs and symptoms may be present.

- Newborn babies with this condition have normal weight and height but may have an open posterior fontanelle or the head may be larger than the normal size.

- Hoarse-sounding cries, drowsiness and decreased muscle tone

- Constipation, enlarged tongue, difficulties with feeding and jaundice

- Decreased body temperature, umbilical hernia and dry skin

- Goiter – It is rare but may occur at a later time in children born with thyroid malfunction

- Delayed growth and intellectual development with IQ 6-15 points lower in severe cases

- Large scale, fine motor skills and coordination problems

- Delayed speaking, decreased attention span and squinting

In older children and adolescents, signs and symptoms include: cold intolerance, fatigue, sleepiness, muscle weakness, delay in growth, and menstrual cycle problems in girls, delayed puberty, constipation, pallor, overweight for height, thick and coarse skin and increased body hair. Delayed relaxation of the reflexes is also common and a slow heartbeat. Goiter or enlargement of the thyroid gland is also present.

In pregnant women, hypothyroidism is often associated with impaired fertility and an increased risk of miscarriage, still-born babies, pre-eclampsia and low-IQ of the offspring.

In infants, you have to be wary of the following:

- Frequent choking

- Yellowing of the white part of the eyes and of the skin, as well. This condition is also called Jaundice and happens when an infant's liver cannot metabolize Bilirubin, a substance that causes red blood cells to be damaged.

- A puffy face

- A protruding and large tongue

- Sleeplessness

- Constipation

And as for children and teens:

- Late development of permanent teeth

- Poor mental development

- Delayed growth, which often results to a short stature

- Delayed puberty or onset of menstruation for teenage girls

Take note that once Hypothyroidism is not treated early, it may worsen and that's why as early as now, you have to make sure that you keep yourself safe from the worsening of this disease. Turn to the next chapter and get to learn about the various ways of combating Hypothyroidism.

Chapter 3: How is Hypothyroidism Diagnosed?

Blood tests are important in the diagnosis of hypothyroidism. It is usually suspected in patients experiencing fatigue, constipation, dry and flaky skin and cold intolerance. If hypothyroidism is diagnosed, then blood levels of thyroid hormones are directly measured and the results are usually very low. In early stages of hypothyroidism, however, T3 and T4 levels in the blood are normal. In this case, the most effective method of measuring hypothyroidism and hyperthyroidism is through the measurement of TSH or thyroid-stimulating hormones.

Laboratory evaluation of TSH is considered the best primary diagnostic test for hypothyroidism. Several weeks later, another TSH level test is needed for further confirmation. In case of other illnesses, levels may be abnormal. However, for people who are confined in the hospital, TSH testing is certainly not encouraged. In cases where TSH levels are elevated, it is an indication that thyroid hormones are not sufficiently produced, therefore T4 tests may be obtained. T3 testing however, is discouraged for hypothyroidism assessment.

If the decrease in thyroid hormone is caused by the pituitary and hypothalamic problems, then it is not surprising if the levels of TSH are abnormally low. As mentioned before, this type of hypothyroidism is known as secondary and tertiary hypothyroidism. In this case, a different method is used for diagnosis. The TRH test can help detect whether the problem is with the hypothalamus or with the pituitary gland. The one who performs this method is an endocrinologist (hormone specialist) and an injection of a TRH hormone is required.

It is important to note though, that blood tests are only effective in detecting the condition of hypothyroidism but it cannot be solely used to detect other underlying causes. Clinical history of the patient, antibody screening, and thyroid scan are the most effective combination of tests to precisely detect the cause of the problem. If suspected with hypothalamic and pituitary problems, an MRI of the brain and other research studies are necessary. These investigations however, are done only on a case to case basis.

If there's no problem detecting hypothyroidism within the thyroid gland, imaging is no longer necessary. If there are thyroid nodules, however, imaging is required.

Pathophysiology of hypothyroidism:

Normal functioning of the tissues inside the human body requires thyroid hormone. Thyroxine or T4 is predominantly secreted by the thyroid gland and this hormone is then converted to T3 or triiodothyronine. Iodothyroonine deiodinase, an enzyme dependent on selenium is responsible for converting thyroxine to triodothyronine in numerous body organs.

The thyroid hormone receptors found in the cell nucleus are bound with triodothyronine and this chemical reaction stimulates the production of proteins and of some specific genes. Furthermore, this process also includes binding with the integrin alpha-v-beta-3 inside the cell membrane. This causes sodium-hydrogen antiporter stimulation, cell growth and blood cells formation.

99.97 percent of thyroid hormone in the blood is bound to protein plasma such as the thyroxine-binding globulin. The only biologically active hormone is the free and unbound thyroid hormone.

When we take a look inside the human body, all thyroid hormones are generated by the thyroid gland. Iodine is extremely important as well as the amino acid tyrosine for this process. The gland absorbs iodine in the blood and mixes it with the molecules of thyroglobulin; then the pituitary gland found in the brain takes control of the process by secreting thyroid-stimulating hormones or TSH. If the process lacks either iodine or TSH, then it automatically results to the low production of thyroid hormones medically termed as hypothyroidism.

To maintain normal thyroid hormone production, the axis hypothalamic-pituitary-thyroid- is maintained as well. The hypothalamus should produce TRH or thyrothropin-releasing hormone to stimulate the production of TSH and TSH should be secreted in the bloodstream to trigger the release of the hormones T3 and T4. If this process is interrupted by any means, production of thyroid hormones is greatly affected. Less TRH results to less TSH and less TSH leads to less thyroid hormones or hypothyroidism.

When a person is pregnant, the thyroid gland increases its size up to 10 percent and this can often result to changes in the physiology of thyroid hormone production. 50 percent increase in the thyroxine production becomes natural as hormonal changes take place inside the body, which in turn increases iodine requirements. This is the reason why it is common for women to acquire hypothyroidism before and after giving birth.

Chapter 4: Risk Factors and Complications

There are several risk factors associated with hypothyroidism. Let us find out who are more at risk in acquiring this condition.

-       Women are more susceptible to having hypothyroidism. Those who have just given birth within the last six months are at risk of acquiring this condition.

-       Women who are already on their senior years especially those who are more than 60 years of age

-       Those people with autoimmune diseases

-       Those who have had undergone thyroid surgery in the past (or partial thyroidectomy)

-       Those who have siblings, relatives, or grandparents who also have autoimmune disease such as diabetes

-       Those who have received radiation treatment on the upper neck or chest are also prone to hypothyroidism.

-       Lastly, those who were once treated with radioactive iodine or anti-thyroid medications are at risk.

Complications:

If hypothyroidism is not treated well, there are several complications that may arise because of that. These complications include:

1.   Goiter – this is the condition wherein the thyroid gland becomes bigger due to the constant stimulation in the gland to release thyroid hormones; another indication of Hashimoto's Thyroiditis. This is generally not life-threatening but it may inhibit discomfort in appearance as well as in breathing and swallowing.

2.   Psychological issues – Hypothyroidism can also cause depression and other mental issues such as intellectual health deterioration especially if the case is severe.

3.   Heart Problems – If a person is diagnosed with hypothyroidism, the presence of LDL or low-density lipoprotein in the blood is increased, thereby resulting to heart problems. Bad cholesterol can occur in people with malfunctioning thyroid glands. It is believed also that even subclinical hypothyroidism can cause increased levels of cholesterol in the body which may slow down one's heartbeat. In more severe cases of hypothyroidism, the heart is enlarged and often fails to pump blood to other parts of the body.

4.   Myxedema – this was already discussed in the previous chapters. Myxedema coma is life-threatening. This can possibly lead to death if not taken cared of properly. This is where immune cells attack and destroy healthy thyroid tissues.

5.   Peripheral neuropathy – If hypothyroidism is not treated properly, this prolonged condition can damage the peripheral nerves especially those at the arms and legs (peripheral nerves are those that carry messages from the central nervous system -brain and the spinal cord- to the rest of the body).

6.   Birth defects – Babies who are born to women with hypothyroidism are prone to certain complications including serious mental deterioration and developmental problems. If this condition is treated at the early stage however, there is a bigger chance of survival and normalized physiological processes.

7.   Infertility – The pituitary gland is responsible for reproduction. If there's a problem with the pituitary, ovulation and fertilization processes are disrupted. Other conditions associated with hypothyroidism such as auto-immune diseases can also impair a person's fertility. For treatment, hormone replacement therapy is not at all effective; further therapies and treatment may be needed to restore a person's impaired fertility.

Chapter 5: Management and Treatment

Treatment and management of hypothyroidism require a life-long process with the exception of other clinical conditions. Here are different methods that can be used in treating hypothyroidism.

1.   Desiccated Animal Thyroid – This desiccated animal thyroid is an animal-based thyroid gland extracted from pigs. It contains numerous hormones including the T3 and T4; calcitonin which is a hormone that regulates the production of calcium levels and is produced in the thyroid gland; and the T1 and T2 that are actually not present in synthetic hormone medications. It was once a popular method of treatment; however, it is no longer supported by the British Thyroid Association while American Professional guidelines do not encourage its application.

2.   Hormone Replacement – People who have been diagnosed with hypothyroidism and those who were concluded to have thyroxine deficiency are treated with artificial and long-acting thyroxine popularly called as the L-thyroxine or levothyroxine. In cases of overt hypothyroidism especially in the young people and healthy patients, it is important to start the full replacement dose immediately. The dosage is adjusted according to the weight of the patient. For the elderly and those with other illnesses or complications, it is advised to start the dosage slowly and gradually to prevent further complications and over-supplementation. People with central hypothyroidism require a higher than average dosage of replacement while

those with subclinical hypothyroidism only requires a minimum dosage.

To ensure that dosage is adequate, series of blood tests are required to monitor thyroxine and TSH or thyroid-stimulating hormone levels. The monitoring is done 4-8 weeks after the initial treatment and change of L-thyroxine dosage. After establishing the replacement dose adequacy, the tests are repeated after 6-12 months depending on the necessity or unless there's a change in the symptoms occurring in the patient's body. Levothyroxine is best taken in 30-60 minutes before breakfast meals and/or 4 hours after the food is digested.

3.   Liothyronine – this is also medically known as the synthetic T3. According to researchers adding Liothyronine to levothyroxine can help regulate the signs and symptoms although there's no evidence to prove such claim as of today. In 2007, British Thyroid Association reported that a combination of T3 and T4 in therapies increases the likelihood of side effects rather than benefits to the patients. They believe that T4 therapy alone is better than these two combined. American Association also seconded this advice because of lack of evidence to pursue otherwise. Furthermore, the effects of liothyronine are short-lived and so the frequency of medication is also increased.

4.   Subclinical   Hypothyroidism   –   Subclinical hypothyroidism is a kind of hypothyroidism but the symptoms are minimal and mild. Often, these signs are not obvious enough. Many people who have this condition do not actually go to their doctors for treatment unless the condition worsens. It is because the treatment for subclinical type of hypothyroidism is not actually that big of a deal to

offer some benefits; nor can it offset the risk of overtreatment. It was found out that in 2007, hormone replacement did not actually give any benefit to people with subclinical hypothyroidism. Both the British and American Associations agree that those people with TSH levels under 10mlU/l do not need any treatment. Treatment and other clinical or medical methods will only be allowed if the TSH levels are elevated more than 10mlU/l.

5.   Myxedema Coma – This condition is actually severe and it is life-threatening, therefore it always requires intensive care. Close monitoring and constant observation is also required and some treatments are applied to correct and regulate abnormalities in the body's temperature, breathing, sodium levels and blood pressure. Mechanical ventilation is also needed as well as vasopressor agents, fluid replacements, corticosteroids and appropriate re-warming.

Vasopressin receptor antagonists and hypertonic saline (salt) solutions are also used to regulate and carefully adjust low sodium levels to normal conditions. In cases where rapid treatment is necessary, both L-thyroxine and liothyronin are administered intravenously. This is applied in cases where the patient is not conscious enough to give consent or is not able to swallow medication safely.

6.   Pregnancy – In case where the patient is pregnant, it is greatly advised that TSH serum should be monitored closely. Within the trimester, TSH levels should be properly regulated to maintain normal levels through the use of levothyroxine. The normal range for the first trimester should be under 2.5mlU/l while both the second and third trimester should be under 3.0mlU/l. Due to the sensitive stage of pregnancy, treatment should be guided totally with

thyroxine and free T4 index. Once pregnancy is confirmed, the levothyroxine dosage is initially elevated.

For women who are trying to get pregnant through natural, assisted or whatever means, thyroid hormone supplementation may still be required even if the TSH levels are normal. This is true for those who have anti-TPO antibodies or if they have a history of miscarriages or hypothyroid condition in the past. Supplementary levothyroxine is also believed to lower the risk of miscarriages and reduce preterm birth.

Lastly, for pregnant women who have subclinical hypothyroidism, thyroid hormone supplementation is strongly suggested. If the person decided not to undergo treatment, close monitoring of the thyroid gland is required. When the test result for anti TPO is not positive, subclinical treatment for hypothyroidism is not recommended.

Chapter 6: Prevention and Screening

Hypothyroidism can certainly be prevented. There are a lot of ways to prevent it from worsening but it is still much better to prevent it from developing.

Prevention:

Although hypothyroidism is fairly common, it can actually be avoided. In some countries, hypothyroidism is reduced through the addition of iodine into the population's diet. Other countries add iodine on their people's diet and it has reduced significant number of hypothyroidism issues especially on children. Such public health measure has been incorporated by each government leaders to effectively eliminate hypothyroidism.

Aside from the promotions on iodine-rich foods incorporated in the dietary menus, many countries that have moderate iodine deficiency have learned to implement universal salt iodization (USI). Today, through the help of World Health Organization, 130 countries have USI and 70% of the populations around the world have access to and receive iodized salt.

In other countries, iodized salt is even used in making bread. Although the world campaign against the use of iodized salts is increasingly effective, iodine deficiency still persists in other Western countries due to other dietary campaigns against iodized salts and their effects on the human body.

Pregnant and lactating women require higher levels of iodine for their offspring; however, they still cannot get enough of it. They are therefore recommended to take 250 µg as instructed. American Thyroid Association also advised that women should all take 150 µg as an oral supplement.

Screening:

Screening is used with TSH and is often performed in newborn babies around the world. The advantage of this method is that early cases and stages of such condition are detected as soon as possible; thus preventing further growth delay and other complications. TSH screening is actually the most common new-born screening method. In case where an underlying cause is unknown or hard to figure out, T4 screening is added to find out the rare causes of neonatal hypothyroidism.

Chapter 7: Eat your way to being healthy

If you cannot let go of your old eating habits and switch to the Gluten Diet easily, don't worry because you would still be able to combat the disease. You just have to be aware of what you eat and learn how to eat only nutritious kinds of food.

But what foods can help you in getting rid of Hypothyroidism? And what should you avoid? Here's what you need to know.

Get rid or eliminate coffee, sugar and carbohydrates

Eat non-starchy foods and vegetables, instead so that your body would be cleansed well and would not rely on sugar to live. Too much Sugar may also cause Hypothyroidism and other diseases such as Diabetes. Your body treats Carbohydrates like sugar and that's why you have to lessen your intake.

Fat can be your friend

Fat is considered as the great balancer of hormonal pathways—which means that you need to have them in your life. After all, if you are going to exercise after consuming some fat, you would be able to burn them away and still be in the right state of your body and in the target weight that you want to be in. You could get healthy fats from avocados, fish, nut butters, nuts, flax, Olive Oil, Ghee, full fat cheese, cottage cheese, yogurt and products made out of coconut milk.

Add Protein in your System

While Gluten is not allowed when it comes to beating Hypothyroidism, other kinds of Proteins are actually recommended for you. Right kinds of protein can be found in whole and grass-fed eggs, fresh fish, grass-fed meats, quinoa, nuts, and nut butters, as well.

Glutathione

More than the number of beauty products filled with Glutathione that have sprouted in the market like mushrooms, Glutathione is actually a healthy anti-oxidant that can be produced by the body by consuming certain kinds of food products, such as: raw eggs, avocados, garlic, squash, spinach, peaches, asparagus, broccoli, and grapefruit. Glutathione helps in producing thyroid hormones and protecting and healing thyroid glands. However, you should also take note that you have to control yourself from eating too much of some of them because they contain Goitrogens, which may interfere with the way your thyroid works. Foods rich in Goitrogen that must be lessened from your diet include:

Kale

- Rutabaga

- Broccoli

- Cauliflower

- Brussels Sprouts

- Millet

- Spinach

- Turnips

- Watercress

- Strawberries

- Peaches

- Peanuts

- Soybeans

- Radish

Take everything in moderation. Don't worry though because you do not have to completely eliminate them from your diet. Once cooked, these food products lose goitrogens. You just have to be careful about eating them raw and in large amounts.

Iodine

As mentioned earlier, Iodine is very important in keeping the body healthy and making sure that you are able to combat Hypothyroidism. It is also great in the prevention of diseases like cretinism, goiter, and mental disabilities, and also aids in the lessening of fatigue, lethargy, weight gain and depression. Iodine is essential in the production of thyroid hormones and that's why you have to include it in your diet. Aside from Iodized salt, which has been proven to reduce the number of patients affected with Hypothyroidism in the United States, other food products that are rich in Iodine include: Dried Seaweed, cod fish, unpeeled baked potato, fish sticks, shrimp, milk, canned tuna with oil, boiled egg, cooked navy beans and cooked turkey breast, as well.

Get rid of Inflammatory Foods

Inflammatory foods or those that cause inflammation inside the body are a big no-no when it comes to fighting Hypothyroidism. People do not usually know which kinds of foods are considered inflammatory and that's why it is very important to check food labels in order for you to understand what it is that you will be eating. Inflammatory foods include:

- **Those with High Trans Fat**. Again, you have to check food labels for this. Trans fat is very inflammable and damages the cells that line your blood vessels which makes it very dangerous.

- **Cheeseburgers**. While they may be delicious and are great comfort foods, research has it that high amount of animal fat causes inflammation. Aside from that, cheeseburgers also cause tissue and gland damage—which might lead to Hypothyroidism instead of getting rid of it.

- **Sugar**. The body cannot break down each and every bit of sugar that you intake and that's why it is essential that you lessen the amount of sugar in your diet.

- **White bread.** This instantly breaks down to sugar as it is full of carbohydrates and as mentioned earlier, you do not need a lot of carbohydrates if you are trying to take care of yourself and trying to get rid of hypothyroidism. White bread makes the body more inflammable and that's not what you'd want to happen.

- **Alcohol**. Aside from the fact that beer is usually made from Barley, too much alcohol makes it easier for bacteria to make their way through your system and damage different tissues and organs. Alcohol also leads to inflammation—you've probably noticed this by the burning sensation you feel while drinking alcohol and just dismissed it as nothing, when in fact, it already damages your system.

- **Omega 6 Fatty Acids**. The difference of these from the healthy Omega 3 Fatty Acids is that they do not do the body good. Omega-6 rich foods include walnuts, vegetable oils and heavy seeds.

- **MSG**. You probably already know that MSG is bad for you and that's why you should cut back on junk foods. MSG can cause a lot of inflammation and may also cause diseases, especially thyroid and kidney related ones and that's why you should cut back on it.

- **Too much milk**. Again, you have to take everything in moderation because too much of anything is never a good thing. Don't drink too much milk especially if you are lactose-intolerant because you will not be able to digest it well.

Detoxify

Going on Detox is not just for those who are trying to get a great figure or are trying to diet just to look good. Detoxification is important for your body and mind to be rejuvenated and refreshed once again. There are so many juice cleanses available right now that you can choose from, or you can choose to make your own if that's more your thing. A combination of Chlorella, Turmeric, Cilantro and Milk Thistle is said to be the best kind of juice cleanse mix that you can take in order to detoxify. You can also juice your choice of fruits and vegetables—what matters is that you drink them for them to work.

Keep these things in mind the next time you go grocery shopping or the next time you eat at a brand new restaurant. Your health should always be your top priority.

Go Gluten Free!

A Gluten-free diet is said to be the most effective, natural way of getting rid of Hypothyroidism. This is a kind of diet that excludes the Protein Gluten from one's daily meals. This is because Gluten is said to be the cause of certain diseases such as Celiac Disease and is also known to damage one's intestines and thyroid glands.

A lot of people find it hard to just leave their old eating habits behind and switch to a Gluten-free kind of life. There's also the thought that one may not get all the nutrients that one's body needs and that are essential to one's growth, such as Iron and Calcium, but Gluten Diet practitioners say that the diet really has done wonders for them and that it can easily help someone to get healthier and be able to fight many diseases such as Hypothyroidism.

Which foods are allowed in this diet?

- Fresh eggs

- Unprocessed seeds, nuts and beans

- Fruits and vegetables

- Dairy products

- Fresh poultry, fish and meat which are not battered, marinated or coated

- Grains such as Buckwheat, Arrowroot, Flax, Corn, Cornmeal, Amaranth, Rice, Millet, Quinoa, Soy, Sorghum, Teff and Tapioca

Which foods should you avoid?

- Wheat

- Rye

- Barley, which means that you should also avoid beer, malt vinegar and malt flavoring that are made from Barley

- Triticale, a mix of wheat and rye

- Durum Flour

- Kamut

- Semolina

- Bulgur

- Farina

- Graham Flour

- Spelt

Aside from these, you should also avoid the foods listed below unless they are labeled as "Gluten-free":

- Pasta

- French Fries

- Gravy

- Candies, cookies and crackers

- Cereals

- Bread

- Salad dressings

- Seasoned potato chips and tortilla chips

- Seasoned rice mixes

- Soy sauce and other sauces

- Vegetables with sauce

- Self-basting poultry

- Processed or canned food such as Luncheon Meat and Corned Beef

- Soup bases and soup

With the right amount of discipline and self-control, you surely will be able to adhere to the Gluten Diet and allow yourself to live a longer and happier life. In the next chapter, you will learn about more ways of letting go of Hypothyroidism by means of what you eat.

Thyroid Gland and Iodine:

Iodine is a common term in the household and in school because it is often associated with iodized salt; but do we really know what iodine is and the role it plays in the human body especially in the thyroid hormone production? We probably imagine iodine as the bright-orange tincture placed on our wounds by a clinic nurse when we get bruises. Believe me, it has the same chemical component but the role it plays inside our body runs far deeper and broader. It is very critical for thyroid hormone production and even a minuscule reduction in the supply can have a large impact on the physiological processes.

With the advent of technology, the growing concern about people not getting enough iodine in their diet plagues a lot of nutritionists, dieticians, scientists and medical doctors. Recently, one statement was released in Newsweek article and a renowned professor said that in the US, iodine deficiency is very rare; however, the Center for Disease Control suggested that it is otherwise and in fact, there were an estimated 2.2 million women who are iodine-deficient.

This portion of the eBook will give you insights as to the importance of iodine in the body. So if you are suffering from hypothyroidism, hyperthyroidism or if you are diagnosed with high blood pressure, fibrocystic breast condition and is under current medication, this portion is for you.

How common is iodine deficiency?

Medical practitioners find iodine issues more and more intriguing. Some of them believe that the case of iodine deficiency is overlooked and downplayed in the United States. In 1920, it was first recognized as a public concern and the government launched programs to add iodine to the salt and flour to ensure that the issue is solved. One out of seven women in the United States was reported to be iodine deficient.

Today, flour is no longer iodized and in the United States, it is only voluntary to iodize the salt and that makes only one-fifth of all the salt produced in the US. Iodine deficiency is starting to rise again. In fact, in the last 4 decades, iodine intake was reduced to 50 percent in North American continent and the statistics remain consistent up to this day. New England Journal defined US iodine status as "marginal" in 2004 and the data collected were based from the data collected by the World Health Organization and International Council for the Control of Iodine Deficiency disorder.

World Health Organization also stated that iodine deficiency is not the greater issue in the US but the iodine-induced hypothyroidism and iodine-induced hyperthyroidism. Both of these health conditions can occur when too much iodine is given very quickly. Practitioners need to prescribe medication or iodine supplements with caution. Iodine levels should be gradually increased when administered.

The reason why iodine-deficiency is often overlooked is because the signs and symptoms are similar with other illnesses and so it may sometimes be confusing. Iodine-deficiency in women was considered a myth by the Nutrition

Survey and 2004 National Health although statistics state that one-third of mature women have reduced or insufficient iodine levels.

Here are some rich sources of iodine:

- Seafood
- Seaweeds or sea vegetables
- Saltwater fish
- Iodized sea salt
- Other foods rich in iodine such as: radishes, dairy products, eggs, onions and watercress.
- Vitamins and mineral supplements also contain iodine.

Why are we iodine deficient?

One-third of the population of the world reside in areas where sources of iodine are relatively low. Iodine is not usually found in top soils and it is often bound tightly in soil particles and that's why crops harvested on land are not always good iodine sources. Evaluation is needed for women who are diagnosed with this condition especially those in the iodine-deficient areas.

The problem does not only lie in the iodine-deficient areas but the more pressing problem is the human actions leading to contaminated surroundings. Our lack of knowledge and ignorance is the main cause why we suffer losses and health risks. Some factors also contribute to iodine deficiency such as over fishing, demonizing of salt, pollution and toxic halide chemicals that replace iodine in our bodies.

Iodophobia:

As we have discussed already, iodine is very important in our body. We need iodine for our normal physiological processes and the lack thereof results to the impairment of thyroid functions. Excessive iodine supply in the body can also elevate thyroid-stimulating hormone levels beyond normal. People who are iodine-replete may have less sensitivity to excessive levels of iodine than those who are iodine-deplete.

The recommended daily allowance of iodine in adults is 150mcg and for lactating women it should be 290mcg a day. Researchers believe that both infants and women will greatly benefit from the increase in RDA especially those with conditions concerning the thyroid, breast and nervous system. In the United States, the current RDA is lower than the upper limit of safety for iodine which is 1,100 mcg. In Europe, it is 600mcg and so iodine deficiency is more common. Japanese people, on the other hand, consume 25 times more than the medium required but no reports of thyroid iodine toxicosis were ever diagnosed.

There are some factors that affect our intake of iodine and these are:

- Iodophobia
- General scarcity of iodine found in the environment
- Environmental and diet changes

How do we treat and test iodine?

They said prevention is better than cure. So to prevent the occurrence of iodine-related conditions and sickness, it is always advised to have regular iodine testing; and if you do have the conditions like hypothyroidism, hyperthyroidism, brain fog, fibrocystic breasts and fatigue, it is always best to detect right away the risks. Iodine is very important as it plays a crucial role in the metabolic processes and the regulation of important hormones such as sex and adrenal hormones.

Self-test is also recommended and it is easily administered using an iodine tincture. Laboratory testing is needed for more advanced and accurate testing though.

What you need to do is to dip a cotton ball (it should be very clean) in a cheap red-tinged Iodine USP tincture which can be bought from any drugstores. Paint a soft skin tissue such as the thigh or inner arm with a 2-inch circle of iodine tincture.

Wait and observe. You will know if you are iodine-replete if the yellow-orange stain disappears and that could take 6 hours. If you are iodine-deficient, the stain will be absorbed very quickly within 1-3 hours.

Chapter 8: Vitamins, Minerals, and Nutrients

Aside from eating the right kind of food, it is also very important for you to take the right kind of supplements and get the best nutrients for you to be able to fight Hypothyroidism well. Here are what you should intake, some foods included, and what you should avoid in order to be able to take care of your thyroid glands better and in order for your body to produce more thyroid hormones:

Stay away from BPA

BPA or Bisphenol A is commonly found in plastic bottles—the kind where you drink juices or teas or even water from. BPA damages your endocrine system and therefore, have bad effects on your thyroid. So, the next time you get thirsty, make it a point to drink only from glass or stainless steel cans. Also, look for the "BPA Free" sign from those plastic bottles to ensure that they are safe to use and drink from.

A Daptogen Supplements

A Daptogen Supplements are known to lower cortisol levels which in turn makes it easy for your thyroid glands to produce more thyroid hormones for you. You need A Daptogen to get rid of Adrenal Fatigue which is also one of the causes of Hypothyroidism. Tulasi, an herb cultivated for medicinal purposes which is also known as Holy Basil, and Ashwagandha or Winter Cherry are great sources of A Daptogen. As these herbs are more commonly found in India than in other parts of the world, taking supplements made out of them would be better than scouring the world to take hold of the herbs yourself.

A need for Selenium

Selenium, although not a very popular mineral, is actually important because it plays a key role in making metabolism faster. Once your metabolism is fast, it means that your body will be able to digest what you have been eating. This way, you're being able to combat Hypothyroidism. Aside from that, it is also known to battle other diseases such as Lung Cancer, Crohn's Disease and Prostate Cancer, as well.

Great sources of Selenium include: Grains, Poultry, Beef, Nuts, Brazil Nuts, Tuna, Herring, Red Snapper and Cod. Whole foods are also good sources of Selenium as the mineral gets dissolved once processing takes place.

Vitamin D

A walk in the sun before 10 am would be good to give your body the amount of Vitamin D that it needs to combat certain kinds of Cancer and Hypothyroidism, as well. Vitamin D3 supplements are also good to give you the Vitamin D that you lack in your system as lack of Vitamin D causes your glands not to produce thyroid hormones that are essential for you.

Iron

Iron is not only good for those who are suffering from Anemia, but is also good for your thyroid glands to produce more thyroid hormones that will help you become strong and will help you say goodbye to Hypothyroidism for good. Aside from taking Iron supplements, you may also eat foods that are rich in Iron, such as egg yolks, red meat, raisins, prunes, spinach, collards, beans, chick peas, lentils, soybeans, artichokes, liver, chicken giblets and turkey, as well. Take Iron along with Vitamin C and you surely will be able to combat the disease even better as Vitamin C is good against inflammation.

Probiotics

Probiotics are more commonly known as good bacteria. Your body needs these as they are the ones who get to fight bad bacteria from taking over your body. Good sources of Probiotics include:

- **Yogurt.** Yogurt is considered as the best source of Probiotics and is also considered as the best substitute for ice cream. Lactobacillus Shirota Strain-filled yogurt products are what you should go for. Aside from being good against Hypothyroidism, yogurt is also good for lessening gas, diarrhea and other kinds of digestive problems.

- **Kefir.** Kefir is a probiotic-filled drink that is said to have originated from Caucasus Mountains of Eurasia. It's almost the same as yogurt but is bubbly, creamy and thick and is good in battling yeast infections.

- **Milk with Probiotics.** There are some milk products that are made with probiotics. You'll know that they are if they are greenish in color and are creamier than your usual kind of milk. It is also commonly known as sweet acidophilus milk. Buttermilk is also known to be rich in probiotics so you can try that, as well.

- **Miso Soup.** Miso is quite popular in Japan and other parts of Asia as a soup made with fish and mustard plus the vegetable bok choi. A bowl of Miso soup contains at least 160 bacteria strains which are about the proper amount that you need each day. It is also low in calories and carbohydrates which make it perfect for someone who is trying to get rid of Hypothyroidism.

- **Sauerkraut.** These days, Sauerkraut is mainly used for sausage dishes and that's why you would not have a hard time trying to find it. Go for unpasteurized Sauerkraut because pasteurization is known to kill good bacteria.

- **Soft Cheese.** Gouda and other kinds of fermented cheese are able to survive in your system for a long time. This means that you will be safe from bad bacteria that damages cells and glands and so you will be able to eliminate the sources of Hypothyroidism.

- **Sourdough Bread.** Sourdough bread is popular for being great in making digestion and metabolism faster. It is also full of Lactobacilli, which are great examples of good bacteria.

- **Sour Pickles.** Pickles are also a good source of probiotics. Go for those that are naturally fermented or those that do not use vinegar in the fermentation process. These pickles also gave metabolic and digestive properties that are truly good for you.

- **Tempeh.** Tempeh is a popular kind of Indonesian Patty that is rich in natural antibiotics that fight bacteria and is also very high in protein. You would not have a hard time liking Tempeh because it is deliciously nutty and smoky and may also taste like a mushroom. You can also marinate Tempeh and add it to other dishes and recipes.

- **Or, you can just try taking Probiotic Supplements.** They are available in liquid, tablet or capsule form and will give you the right amount of Probiotics that you need.

Chapter 9: Thyroid Stimulating Exercises

Contrary to popular belief, there are actually some exercises that patients who suffer from Hypothyroidism can do. Just because you are suffering from Hypothyroidism does not mean that you can no longer workout or use your body for physical activities. Thinking this way would just worsen your disease.

Walking Daily

You'd be surprised to know how much walking contributes to your well-being. If you need to go somewhere and it's not far away from home, why not try walking instead of taking a can or riding other forms of public transport? Aside from the fact that you will be able to save some money, walking is simple and will also help you appreciate the beauty of your surroundings even better. Walking for around 20 to 40 minutes per day is already good to combat Hypothyroidism— it helps you lose weight and makes your metabolism faster. It also lets your thyroid glands work at an optimal rate.

Jogging

You don't need to do it professionally. Do it early in the morning or at night, upon coming home. You can do it in your own backyard if you want or use your village or the nearby park to jog. What's important is that you do it once or twice a week so that you'd get to burn all the extra fats that you have accumulated and so that your body will feel refreshed.

Circuit Training

Circuit Training is also proven to help reduce the risk of Hypothyroidism. Circuit Training also helps lower insulin levels, which in turn protects you against Diabetes. Some examples of these exercises include push-ups, lunges, curl-ups, bench presses, and sit ups for a couple of repetitions. If you do not like to go to the gym, then you can also do the exercises at the comforts of your own home. Rest a bit to catch your breath then do them again. You can devote at least 10 to 20 minutes of your day to Circuit Training and you will be alright.

Get to know your Acupressure Points

Devoting a bit of your time to massage or relax different Acupressure Points in your body would do wonders for your system when it comes to battling Hypothyroidism. You can do these for at least 2 to 5 times daily for them to work better. Some examples include:

- **Neck-Press.** Sit down and close your eyes and interlace your hands behind your neck, or on your nape. Bow your head down a bit and just relax. This way, you will be able to stretch your neck muscles. Then, bring your elbows together in front of you and compress the sides of your neck using your hands. Raise your head as you stretch gently and inhale and exhale as you relax. Repeat the exercise for at least 2 minutes.

- **K 27.** K 27 is known as both sides of your sternum. Just take long, deep breaths and turn your head from side to side. Allow yourself to feel how your neck region relaxes and just go and breathe deeply as you hold the K27 spots. Tilt your head up as you inhale, and down as you exhale and visualize the things that you want to have or the things you want to do someday. This is a good way of meditating, as well so not only do you help your body, you also get to clear your mind of its worries.

- **Temples.** Use your index and middle finger to massage your temples. Sit down, relax and massage both temples in circular motions. These will easily help you ease the pain that you are feeling and would also help you relax.

Chapter 10: Alternative Hypothyroidism Treatments

Alternative medicine is often used to treat illnesses and other medical conditions. Practitioners believe that poor health can be resolved better with alternative treatments rather than simply treating and relieving the signs and symptoms. In the case of hypothyroidism, alternative treatments usually prevent the development of full-blown thyroid disease by reversing the suboptimal functioning of the thyroid gland. However, it is important to note that the success of alternative medicine depends on the extent of autoimmune anti-bodies already present in the body and how early the intervention and treatment was started.

The origin of many diseases and medical conditions is poor nutrition so the first thing to do is to ensure that proper and healthy diet is observed for people with hypothyroidism. This may not resolve the condition but it can prevent it from worsening. Ensure that various nutrients are taken in like folic acid, selenium and iodine. Supplement is also vital with medical grade to optimize the levels of nutrition with balanced diet.

Aside from nutrition, stress is another huge factor in the development of hypothyroidism. For people with this condition, it is important to identify the causes of stress and find strategies and techniques to better combat these stressors.

So here are the guidelines that people with hypothyroidism should follow to ensure maximum health benefits and prevent further health decline. Commitment to this healthy regimen and self-care is very important.

These are:

- Consumption of seeds, nuts and whole grains that are naturally rich in Vitamin B complex
- Consumption of foods rich in iodine such as root vegetables, seaweed, fish, and vegetables
- Daily exercise for at least 30-60 minutes or at least 4 times a week
- Deep breathing exercises that can be practiced daily through visualization and meditation for relaxation
- Exposure to the sun for at least 15 minutes in Northern climate; this is crucial in obtaining sufficient Vitamin D levels. Vitamin D helps facilitate cell metabolism and supports the immune system. You should discuss this treatment option with a medicine practitioner especially during winter seasons.
- Emotional issues should be dealt with. Women should use their voices more often or better yet voice out their feelings and frustrations. Note that suppressing their voices especially when they feel bad can cause their throat to accumulate "trapped voices"; this will eventually lead to thyroid malfunction when a woman reaches the peri-menopausal stage. Talk more to reduce thyroid stress.
- Other alternative medicines should be carefully considered as well such as acupuncture, homeopathic medicine, traditional Chinese medicine, osteopathy, naturopathic medicine and biofeedback.

Most often, these guidelines plus other alternative medicines that directly treat thyroid malfunction and help in correcting nutritional imbalances and emotional stress restores normal thyroid function totally.

Natural Solutions for the Thyroid:

Natural remedies for hypothyroidism include minerals, herbs and plants and they help strengthen the thyroid gland. There are reports that women who tried natural remedies felt so much better even without the benefits and help from over-the-counter medicines and medical intervention. This proves that natural solutions for thyroid problems are effective when properly and conscientiously observed by the person.

There's one story that can attest to the effectiveness of these natural remedies. The woman's name is Alexa and she was diagnosed with hypothyroidism. She is still at her early thirties and she complains of weight gain, and itchy and dry skin. Medical practitioners disregarded the issue and they didn't think it was something to worry about. They just thought that Alexa gained weight because of the cold climate in the north and her dry and itchy skin is a common issue because of the cold. She just shrugged it off and applied moisturizer on her skin and lessened her food intake.

One day, Alexa experienced so much itchiness and it became unbearable. That's the time she realized that something was not right. Her mother has a medical condition – hypothyroidism- and she had been taking prescriptions for years.

Alexa then went back to the doctor and her doctor saw that her thyroid gland is malfunctioning. They prescribed medicines and supplements but Alexa didn't feel satisfied with the prescriptions. What she did was look for natural remedies and she did a lot of research. She looked for an alternative medicine practitioner and for six months she followed the natural approach. Alexa soon found that natural remedies worked better for her than prescriptions.

Minerals and Plants for your Thyroid:

Thyroid is considered as the master gland inside the human body. It usually has a role to play in every part and systems of our body. When the hormones produced by the thyroid are not sufficient, all the other internal processes will be affected and imbalanced as well. Likewise, if there are any imbalances in the internal processes such as the adrenal system, thyroid is also affected.

Here are some benefits from minerals and plants:

- Minerals and plants provide a boost of energy which is good for people with hypothyroidism as they often complain of weight gain and fatigue.
- They also help in the regulation of cell metabolism and in the maintenance of thyroid hormones production.
- Natural remedies also provide benefits and support even without the aid of prescriptions and the effects can be expected to last for the rest of your life.

Plants and minerals are great alternatives for mild cases of hypothyroidism but in more common cases, these can provide good support even if the person is taking medical prescriptions. Natural approach may even help reduce the medical intervention and prescriptions given to the patient. Just remember that there are only 2 most important nutrients for the thyroid gland to function normally; these are selenium and iodine.

Aside from iodine and selenium, other plants and minerals have the ability to adapt to what the body needs. They provide what is lacking in your body. Interestingly, there are some plants that can copy what our body can do if it is functioning normally. This process is called the "adaptogenic effect". This is where the minerals and plant nutrients act as support and allow our body to use what it needs despite not knowing what the problem is.

Natural remedies should be carefully checked and you need to constantly seek the advice of your chosen alternative medicine practitioner. You should always inform him of everything that you take. If there are any changes, do not hesitate to report it so you can see what to do right away. Take good care of yourself and follow a strict healthy diet to ensure a lifetime of feeling good. Learn to cope with stress by practicing yoga and meditation. Practice breathing exercises and stretch your muscles as often as possible.

Symptoms and signs of hypothyroidism clearly vary from one person to another. When you are diagnosed with this condition you ought to know what options you have. This way, you can help yourself and you can choose what's best for you. Your health will always depend on you. You are the only one who is responsible for your body so take good care of it.

Other reminders:

Aside from what was discussed in earlier chapters, here are some of the other things that you should keep in mind for you to be able to battle your disease.

Eliminate Stress

Stress causes you to feel bad about yourself, does not put your mind at ease, and also is one of the reasons why you get to suffer from some diseases such as Hypothyroidism because it causes your adrenal and thyroid glands to be exhausted. In order to eliminate stress, you should:

- **Try Meditation**. Go to a quiet place, think of a mantra, repeat it over and over again, and then make sure that you get to understand that it is true. For example, say "I can do this" or "I can get rid of this disease", and believe in it for it to be true. The power of positive thinking would really do you wonders so do not underestimate it.

- **Get an ample amount of sleep**. Sleeping for 6 to 8 hours each night, even if you are already an adult, is essential to help you become healthy and in top shape. If you get the right amount of sleep, you'd feel better about yourself and about the day that you are going to embark on. Getting the right amount of sleep equals happiness, so why would you deprive yourself of sleep?

- **Write your feelings down.** Creating a blog or writing on a journal always helps to make you feel better about yourself because you will be able to put your feelings out and let go of whatever it is that's bothering you. This way, you will be able to understand yourself better and get a clear mind when it comes to knowing that you will be able to battle the disease and let go of it—just as long as you believe that you can.

- **Do what you love.** It's much like a cliché, but doing what you love can do you wonders. When you know that you are doing things that people say you cannot do, or that are deemed as stupid, even if they are not, would surely make you feel better about yourself and would help lessen the stress in your life.

Drink lots of water

Another fact of life that most people take for granted is the fact that water is important to good health. It is also a given fact that drinking water is essential for those who have thyroid problems or thyroid related diseases. Aside from the traditional 8 glasses a day, you'd have to drink another glass for each pound that you want to lose.

Drink Green Tea

Research has it that aside from being able to cleanse your system, Green Tea is also good in making you more adept in exercising and in helping you feel better about yourself while exercising. And, it also calms you down which makes you feel less stressed and more motivated.

Remove Silver Fillings

If you've gotten treatment or Pasta for your teeth, you may have gotten silver fillings without being aware of it. These are also called Amalgam Fillings and may have high amounts of mercury which are dangerous to the body. It would be good to ask your dentist about what's in your Pasta before getting one, and if you already have one, then look for a dentist that offers Amalgam-free types of Pasta so that you will be safer. Amalgam also disrupts thyroid production and that's why you have to get rid of it.

And, Try Heat Therapy

Going to the sauna, taking a hot shower, or relaxing in a hot spring is great not only because they are able to help you relax and feel calmer, they are also able to eliminate stored toxins. It's important to get rid of the body's stored toxins as these only blocks the production of thyroid hormones which then causes Hypothyroidism.

Conclusion

Thank you again for purchasing this book!

I hope this book was able to help you to understand what Hypothyroidism is all about, how you will know that you have the disease and what to do to get rid of it.

The next step is to not only read and keep this book, but to actually try what is written in here. If you want to let go of your disease, then you should believe that you can and you should do whatever you can to let go of it and not let it take over your life. With the help of this book, you certainly can do it.

Finally, if you enjoyed this book, please take the time to share your thoughts and post a review on Amazon. We do our best to reach out to readers and provide the best value we can. Your positive review will help us achieve that. It'd be greatly appreciated!

Thank you and good luck!

Check Out My Other Books

Below you'll find some of my other popular books that are popular on Amazon and Kindle as well. Simply click on the links below to check them out. Alternatively, you can visit my author page on Amazon to see other work done by me.

Coconut Oil for Easy Weight Loss: A Step by Step Guide for Using Virgin Coconut Oil for Quick and Easy Weight Loss

http://www.amazon.com/Coconut-Oil-Easy-Weight-Loss-ebook/dp/B00JG8H8DE

Superfoods that Kickstart Your Weight Loss Learn How to Use 30 Superfoods to Boost Weight Loss, Immunity and to Live a Healthier Lifestyle

http://www.amazon.com/Superfoods-that-Kickstart-Your-Weight-ebook/dp/B00JNAPM9M

Carrier Oils for Beginners: Discover the Characteristics and Beauty and Health Benefits of Carrier Oils For mixing Aromatherapy Essential Oils

http://www.amazon.com/Carrier-Oils-Beginners-Characteristics-Aromatherapy-ebook/dp/B00K88GI2S

Natural Homemade Cleaning Recipes For Beginners: Essential Oil Recipes For Household Cleaning, Laundry & Toxic Free Living

http://www.amazon.com/Natural-Homemade-Cleaning-Recipes-Beginners-ebook/dp/B00K87UBQI

The Best Secrets of Natural Remedies: The Ultimate Guide to Natural Remedies to Prevent and Cure Illnesses, Cold and Flu for Your Family

http://www.amazon.com/Best-Secrets-Natural-Remedies-Illnesses-ebook/dp/B00JNDCOCM

The Hypothyroidism Handbook:An Everyday Guide to Natural Solutions of living with Hypothyroidism including increased energy, lasting weight loss, and general well-being

http://www.amazon.com/Hypothyroidism-Handbook-Solutions-including-increased-ebook/dp/B00JNIGIV0

The Hyperthyroidism Handbook: An Everyday Guide to Natural Solutions of Living with Hyperthyroidism including Weight Gain, Increased Energy and General Well-being

http://www.amazon.com/Hyperthyroidism-Handbook-Solutions-including-Hypothyroidism-ebook/dp/B00JOHU5SM

Essential Oils & Weight Loss for Beginners: Ultimate Guide to Losing Weight, Increasing Energy, Balancing Metabolism & Appetite Using Essential Oils & Aromatherapy

http://www.amazon.com/Essential-Oils-Weight-Loss-Beginners-ebook/dp/B00JOFOWP6

Top Essential Oil Recipes: A Recipe Guide Of Natural, Non-Toxic Aromatherapy & Essential Oils for Healing Common Ailments, Beauty, Stress & Anxiety

http://www.amazon.com/Top-Essential-Oil-Recipes-Aromatherapy-ebook/dp/B00JY434E2

Soap Making For Beginners: A Guide to Making Natural Homemade Soaps from Scratch, Includes Recipes and Step by Step Processes for Making Soaps

http://www.amazon.com/Soap-Making-Beginners-Homemade-Processes-ebook/dp/B00JYKH75I

Body Butters For Beginners: Proven Secrets To Making All Natural Body Butters For Rejuvenating And Hydrating Your Skin

http://www.amazon.com/Body-Butters-Beginners-Rejuvenating-Hydrating-ebook/dp/B00K6LVV6A

Apple Cider Vinegar For Beginners: Proven Secrets Using Apple Cider Vinegar For Health, Weight Loss, and Skin Care

http://www.amazon.com/Apple-Cider-Vinegar-Beginners-Aromatherapy-ebook/dp/B00K6YY6HI

Homemade Body Scrubs & Masks For Beginners: 50 Proven All Natural, Easy Recipes For Body & Facial Masks To Exfoliate Nourish, & Care For Your Skin

http://www.amazon.com/Homemade-Body-Scrubs-Masks-Beginners-ebook/dp/B00K79D4SY

Essential Oils Box Set #1: Essential Oils & Weight Loss For Beginners (Ultimate Guide to Losing Weight, Increasing Energy, Balancing Metabolism & Appetite Using Essential Oils & Aromatherapy) + Top Essential Oil Recipes (A Recipe Guide of Natural, Non-Toxic Aromatherapy & Essential Oils for Healing Common Ailments, Beauty, Stress & Anxiety)

http://www.amazon.com/ESSENTIAL-OILS-BOX-SET-Aromatherapy-ebook/dp/B00K7Q8HRK

Essential Oils Box Set #2: Essential Oils & Weight Loss For Beginners (Ultimate Guide to Losing Weight, Increasing Energy, Balancing Metabolism & Appetite Using Essential Oils & Aromatherapy) + Top Essential Oil Recipes (A Recipe Guide of Natural, Non-Toxic Aromatherapy & Essential Oils for Healing Common Ailments, Beauty, Stress & Anxiety)

http://www.amazon.com/ESSENTIAL-OILS-BOX-SET-Aromatherapy-ebook/dp/B00K7Q8HRK

Box Set#3: Coconut Oil for Easy Weight Loss(A Step by Step Guide for Using Virgin Coconut Oil for Quick and Easy Weight Loss) + Apple Cider Vinegar(Proven Secrets Using Apple Cider Vinegar for Health, Weight Loss, and Skin Care)

http://www.amazon.com/Box-Set-Beginners-Aromatherapy-Essential-ebook/dp/B00K9TEGUW

Box Set #4: Body butters For Beginners(Proven Secrets To Making All Natural Body Butters For Rejuvenating And Hydrating Your Skin) & Top Essential Oil Recipes: A Recipe Guide Of Natural, Non-Toxic Aromatherapy & Essential Oils for Healing Common Ailments, Beauty, Stress & Anxiety

http://www.amazon.com/Box-Set-Butters-Beginners-Essential-ebook/dp/B00KA02F4Y

Box Set #5: Soap Making For Beginners(A Guide to Making Natural Homemade Soaps from Scratch, Includes Recipes and Step by Step Processes for Making Soaps) + Homemade Body Scrubs & Masks For Beginners(50 Proven All Natural, Easy Recipes For Body Scrub & Facial Masks To Efoliate, Nourish, & Care For Your Skin)

http://www.amazon.com/Box-Set-Beginners-Homemade-Recipes-ebook/dp/B00K9U3I2I

Box Set #6: Body Butters for Beginners (Proven Secrets To Making All Natural Body Butters For Rejuvenating And Hydrating Your Skin) +Homemade Body Scrubs & Masks For Beginners(50 Proven All Natural, Easy Recipes For Body Scrub & Facial Masks To Exfoliate, Nourish, & Care For Your Skin)

http://www.amazon.com/Box-Set-Beginners-Exfoliating-Moisturizing-ebook/dp/B00K9U3Y4O

Box Set #7: TOP ESSENTIAL OILS(A Recipe Guide Of Natural, Non-Toxic Aromatherapy & Essential Oils For Healing, Common Ailments, Beauty, Stress & Anxiety) & THE BEST SECRETS OF NATURAL REMEDIES(The Ultimate Guide to Natural Remedies to Prevent and Cure Illnesses, Cold and Flu for Your Family)

http://www.amazon.com/BOX-SET-Essential-Recipes-Remedies-ebook/dp/B00K9WPMQG

Box Set #8: NATURAL HOMEMADE CLEANING RECIPES FOR BEGINNERS (Essential Oil Recipes for Household Cleaning, Laundry & Toxic Free Living) + TOP ESSENTIAL OILS(A Recipe Guide Of Natural, Non-Toxic Aromatherapy & Essential Oils For Healing, Common Ailments, Beauty, Stress & Anxiety)

http://www.amazon.com/BOX-SET-Beginners-Essential-Aromatherapy-ebook/dp/B00KAMNGBS

Box Set #9: Essential Oils & Weight Loss for Beginners (Ultimate Guide to Losing Weight, Increasing Energy, Balancing Metabolism & Appetite Using Essential Oils & Aromatherapy) + Carrier Oils for Beginners (Discover the Characteristics and Beauty and Health Benefits of Carrier Oils for Mixing Aromatherapy Essential Oils) http://www.amazon.com/BOX-SET-Essential-Beginners-Aromatherapy-ebook/dp/B00KAODL6Q

BOX SET #10: THE HYPERTHYROIDISM HANDBOOK (An Everyday Guide to Natural Solutions of Living with Hyperthyroidism including Weight Gain, Increased Energy and General Well-being) + THE HYPOTHYROIDISM HANDBOOK (Everyday Guide to Natural Solutions of Living With Hypothyroidism Including Increased Energy, Lasting Weight Loss, and General Well-Being)

http://www.amazon.com/BOX-SET-10-Hyperthyroidism-Hypothyroidism-ebook/dp/B00KAKMSBY

BOX SET #11: CARRIER OILS FOR BEGINNERS (Discover the Characteristics and Beauty and Health Benefits of Carrier Oils for Mixing Aromatherapy Essential Oils) + Essential Oils & Aromatherapy for Beginners (Secrets to Beauty, Health and Weight Loss Using Proven Essential Oil and Aromatherapy Recipes

http://www.amazon.com/BOX-SET-Beginners-Essential-Aromatherapy-ebook/dp/B00KAONEQ8

BOX SET 12: ESSENTIAL OILS & WEIGHT LOSS FOR BEGINNERS: (Ultimate Guide to Losing Weight, Increasing Energy, Balancing Metabolism & Appetite Using Essential Oils & Aromatherapy) + TOP ESSENTIAL OIL RECIPES (A Recipe Guide of Natural, Non-Toxic Aromatherapy & Essential Oils for Healing Common Ailments, Beauty, Stress & Anxiety) + CARRIER OILS FOR BEGINNERS (Discover the Characteristics & Beauty & Health Benefits of Carrier Oils for Mixing Aromatherapy Essential Oils) + ESSENTIAL OILS & AROMATHERAPY FOR BEGINNERS (Secrets to Beauty & weight Loss Using Proven Essential Oil & Aromatherapy Recipes) + NATURAL HOMEMADE CLEANING RECIPES FOR BEGINNERS (Essential Oil

Recipes for Household Cleaning, Laundry & Toxic Free Living)

http://www.amazon.com/BOX-SET-12-Essential-Aromatherapy-ebook/dp/B00KCBCHE4

BOX SET #13: SUPERFOODS THAT KICKSTART YOUR WEIGHT LOSS (Learn How to Use 30 Superfoods to Boost Weight Loss, Immunity and to Live a Healthier Lifestyle) + ESSENTIAL OILS & AROMATHERAPY FOR BEGINNERS (Secrets to Beauty, Health and Weight Loss Using Proven Essential Oil and Aromatherapy Recipes) + BODY BUTTERS FOR BEGINNERS (Proven Secrets To Making All Natural Body Butters For Rejuvenating And Hydrating Your Skin) + SOAP MAKING FOR BEGINNERS (A Guide to Making Natural Homemade Soaps from Scratch, Includes Recipes and Step by Step Processes for Making Soaps) + HOMEMADE BODY SCRUBS FOR BEGINNERS (50 Proven All Natural, Easy Recipes For Body Scrub & Facial Masks To Exfoliate, Nourish, & Care For Your Skin)

http://www.amazon.com/BOX-SET-Superfoods-Kickstart-Aromatherapy-ebook/dp/B00KC8G6DK/

BOX SET 14: Essential Oils & Weight Loss for Beginners (Ultimate Guide to Losing Weight, Increasing Energy, Balancing Metabolism & Appetite Using Essential Oils & Aromatherapy) + Apple Cider Vinegar for Beginners (Proven Secrets Using Apple Cider Vinegar for Health, Weight Loss, and Skin Care) + Body Butters For Beginners (Proven Secrets To Making All Natural Body Butters For Rejuvenating And Hydrating Your Skin)
+ Homemade Body Scrubs & Masks for Beginners (50 Proven All Natural, Easy Recipes for Body Scrub & Facial Masks to Exfoliate, Nourish, & Care for Your Skin) + Coconut Oil for Easy Weight Loss (A Step by Step Guide for Using Virgin Coconut Oil for Quick and Easy Weight Loss)

http://www.amazon.com/BOX-SET-Essential-Beginners-Aromatherapy-ebook/dp/B00KEDO68U

If the links do not work, for whatever reason, you can simply search for these titles on the Amazon website to find them.